NATURAL REMEDIES TO FIGHT HYPERTENSION

50 PLUS REMEDIES TO COMBAT HIGH BLOOD PRESSURE NATURALLY

TABLE OF CONTENT

1. CHAPTER I. INTRODUCTION-HYPERTENSION-WHAT IS IT?

Hypertension which is commonly referred to as HTN and high blood pressure and sometimes it is called arterial hypertension, is a common medical condition that puts pressure on the heart due to elevated pressure of blood in the arteries. Blood pressure can be measured by the systolic and diastolic pressure depending upon the contraction and relaxation of the heart muscles.

HTN can either be primary or secondary depending upon the causes leading to it. Primary hypertensive cases make up to around 90 to 95 percent and are characterized by high blood pressure with no obvious medical underlying causes behind. While the remaining 5 to 10 percent belong to secondary hypertension and in this many underlying conditions may be prevalent and are responsible for its progression which may include heart or endocrine problems, Cushing syndrome, preeclampsia, hyperparathyroidism, arterial or kidney problems, etc.

There may not be any visible symptoms most of the time which could be misleading and could only be diagnosed after a thorough medical checkup. Due to not being aware of their condition for a long period of time, people can develop kidney, heart, or arterial problems. Some of the signs and symptoms of dangerous type of HTN which is also known as malignant hypertension may include severe headache, nausea, vomiting, visionary changes, confusion and nose bleed.

There are many causes which may play a part in the development and progression of this health problem which may include family history, diabetes, unhealthy diet, high intake of dietary sodium, excess alcohol intake, stress, anxiety, smoking, etc. If this condition is left uncontrolled and untreated it may start to show signs and symptoms of many health concerns, conditions and chronic diseases such as heart failure, kidney diseases, stroke and heart attack. In other words, it leads to reduced life expectancy.

Many factors play a role in affecting blood pressure negatively which may include water retention, kidney problems, diseased blood vessels, nervous system problems, hormonal imbalance, etc. Blood pressure needed to be tested regularly. Home based kits are easier to handle, inexpensive and more practical for regular checkup and could be utilized by the whole family. Learn the technique through a professional guidance before opting for home use.

The goal of treatment must be to reduce blood pressure and to decrease chances of risk factors linked with several chronic diseases. Lifestyle changes in addition to medications may be needed. Eating a heart friendly diet, increasing physical activity, quitting smoking and other unhealthy habits, reducing tension, stress, anxiety and depression level, limiting alcohol and salt intake, maintaining ideal body weight are few of the many factors that influences blood pressure and proper management may help in lessening the chances of onset of this condition.

Uncontrolled hypertension may lead to increased risk factors leading to serious health problems, therefore timely action is needed and total commitment to follow the treatment as well as complete change of lifestyle patterns may at times be recommended. Healthy lifestyle changes in a family may not only be beneficial for a single person diagnosed with this problem but will prove to be beneficial for many associated with that person.

Quitting smoking, reducing salt intake, limiting alcohol consumption, healthy dietary changes and increased physical activity are few of the many beneficial lifestyle changes that may not only help in treating the problem from grass root level but may be beneficial in preventing its occurrence in a family. Research has shown that some herbs, supplements and relaxation techniques can work well in the treatment process to combat this condition in addition to conventional treatment.

This disease affects so many people that prescription medications have been developed to treat it. In addition to this, a number of alternative and complementing therapies could be used. Some alternative therapies and natural medicines have been known to help reduce high blood pressure to some extent.

2. CHAPTER II. SIGNS AND SYMPTOMS OF HYPERTENSION

High blood pressure is rarely accompanied by any signs and symptoms initially. Health care screening may be needed to identify this health problem. Small numbers of people do report of certain symptoms which may include headache, light headedness, tinnitus, vertigo, fainting episodes, altered vision, etc. Many of these symptoms may be due to the related anxiety associated with this problem rather than HTN itself.

After carrying out the physical examination, hypertension could be detected due to the presence of hypertensive retinopathy by examining the optic fundus by the use of ophthalmoscopy. These findings may be helpful in determining for how long a person has been affected by this disease. Hypertensive retinopathy and its severity are being graded from I to IV, although it is difficult to distinguish between the mild types.

Some signs and symptoms may also suggest secondary type of hypertension that may be linked to an identifiable cause or disease such as endocrine or kidney disease. Cushing's syndrome that may be one of the causes behind could show signs and symptoms of stretch marks, moon face, a buffalo hump, glucose intolerance, obesity, etc. Severely elevated hypertension may lead to hypertensive crises and many complications and risk factors are associated with this kind of elevation.

Many signs and symptoms may suggest severe elevation of hypertension and people may report headache and dizziness. As the condition may become more serious and start to deteriorate, additional symptoms may become more evident which may include breathlessness, visual deterioration, and feeling of malaise, heart failure or renal failure.

Severely high blood pressure could lead to emergency crises as it is a sign of malignant hypertension and directly responsible in damaging the body organs which may include brain, liver, kidney and heart. This can lead to brain swelling and hypertensive encephalopathy. The signs and symptoms of these may be indicated by chest pain which may lead to myocardial infarction or sometimes to the tearing of the inner wall of the aorta also called aorta dissection.

Pulmonary edema is characterized by signs and symptoms such as cough, breathlessness, blood stained sputum, swelling of the lung tissues, etc. Kidney function may deteriorate rapidly. Rapid reduction of hypertension may be required to protect the body organs from ongoing damage. Usually medications are required during hypertensive emergencies.

3. CHAPTER III. CAUSES OF HYPERTENSION

Essential or primary hypertension is the most common type of high blood pressure accounting for around 90 to 95 % of all the reported cases. High blood pressure risk may increase with progression in age. Interaction of genes and innumerable environmental factors may leave their influences to affect blood pressure and are complex to understand.

Factors influencing in reducing the blood pressure may include reduced intake of dietary salt, low fat intake, increased intake of fruits, increased physical activity, ideal body weight maintenance, limiting intake of alcohol, relaxation techniques, reducing stress level, deep breathing techniques, etc. Reducing the anxiety level and increasing physical activity may also play a role in reducing high blood pressure.

Many events occurring early in life may impact and leave its influences contributing to the onset of hypertension later in life such as low birth weight and maternal smoking.

Identifiable causes may be behind secondary hypertension which may include renal disease and endocrine problems such as Cushing's syndrome, hypothyroidism, hyperthyroidism, acromegaly, hyperaldosteronism, hyperparathyroidism and pheochromocytoma. Several other causes may include sleep apnea, obesity, pregnancy, and excess consumption of licorice, coarctation of the aorta and use of certain medications, herbs and drugs.

The diagnosis is based on persistent increase in blood pressure. Initial assessment is based on physical examination and medical history. Several readings may be required for more than once before the final diagnosis. After diagnosis, identification of risk factors, underlying causes and associated symptoms may be looked into. Essential or primary hypertension is more common among the adolescents and multiple risk factors may be involved which may include obesity, diet genetics, etc.

4. CHAPTER 1V. TREATMENT OF HYPERTENSION

Treatment may involve overall lifestyle changes in addition to medication and dietary changes. If you are over-weight then you may require shedding off all the extra pounds through a well-planned dietary regimen and by increasing the physical activity. Increasing physical activity not only helps in achieving your target ideal body weight but is also beneficial in keeping the overall body systems in peak working condition.

Natural means of prevention and treatment aids in reducing the drug dependency and to avoid innumerable and unavoidable side effects attached with these. Drug dependency and dosage can be delayed and reduced if proper management of natural means is handled effectively. Dietary regimen must meet the modifications needed and a more adapted version of a low sodium diet may be required and needed to be planned to meet and suit each individual needs and requirements.

A dash diet is usually a low sodium diet which is high in potassium, calcium, magnesium and protein. It is rich in whole grains, nuts, fish, poultry, vegetables and fruits. This kind of diet is helpful in reducing the blood pressure and major feature of this kind of diet plan is to limit intake of dietary sodium. Reducing the stress level is another beneficial treatment regimen and learning the technique of relaxation through means of meditation, aromatherapy, yoga, etc. may be needed.

Exercise regimen program for the treatment purpose may include isometric resistance exercise, resistance exercise, aerobic exercise and device guided breathing exercise. Meditation may depend on individual need and several risk factors may be attached with individualized cases.

If drug treatment has been initiated then monitoring of the blood pressure on regular basis and looking for any kind of side effects is needed. Majority of the people need more than one kind of drug and your physician may be your best guide so that you do not take wrong or unacceptable combinations. Reducing the blood pressure in hypertensive cases helps in increasing the life expectancy.

In the year 2000 a study conducted revealed that around 26 % of the world adult population had hypertension which comes to nearly one billion people. Different regions show different patterns, some showing as low as 5 % while others showing as high as 70 %. India had the lowest incidence level while Poland had the highest.

May be this is because the Indian population mainly depends to a great extent on the consumption of plant sources of food while rest of the world's dependency on food sources largely come through the animal sources. Animal sources of foods are high in cholesterol as well as saturated fat while plant based food is cholesterol and saturated fat free with only few exceptions which may include coconut oil.

Coconut is one of the rare plant based sources of saturated fat but has been found to be beneficial for overall health and especially good for the health of the heart. High dietary consumption of saturated fats has been linked to heart problems including high blood pressure.

5. CHAPTER V. FIFTY NATURAL REMEDIES FOR HYPERTENSION

1. Make *garlic* a part of your regular meal as it helps in preventing plaque buildup in the arteries, decrease blood clotting and helps in widening the arteries.

2. *Hawthorn berries* have also been found to be beneficial in providing protection from arterial problems and consequently to hypertension.

3. *Ginko biloba* has been known to dilate the arteries and improving blood circulation and reducing chances of developing hypertension.

4. If the problem of hypertension is stress related than you may make use of *valerian, passion flower, lime flower and lemon balm* as these possess sedative properties which help in reducing the stress and anxiety level and do not possess any kind of side effects. Valerian may also help in smoothening of the muscles that line the artery walls and helps in preventing constricting.

5. Use of *angelica* and *horseradish* may also be helpful.

6. *Sapodilla (cheeko)* has also been found to be beneficial.

7. Eat *fish* and make use of fish oil regularly.

8.   Eat *celery* as it has been used historically to lower the blood pressure.

9.   Eat lots of *broccoli* as it is a rich source of calcium and magnesium.

10.   *Beet root* and beet root juice has been found to be effective in bringing rapid reduction in hypertension naturally

11.   Eating a handful of *raw almonds* on a daily basis is also recommended as these are a rich source of monounsaturated fats and helps in lowering the serum cholesterol level, lowers blood pressure and reduce arterial inflammation. These are also beneficial in reducing weight and promote healthy circulation in the body. These are considered powerful super foods of cardiovascular.

12.   *Cayenne pepper* is one of the fastest blood pressures reducing food and helps in expanding the blood vessels to bring improvement in the blood flow. It increases the rate of blood flow throughout the body. You may mix a little in honey for regular use to alleviate high blood pressure.

13.   *Coconut water* has also been found to be helpful significantly to lower your blood pressure levels as it is rich in potassium and electrolytes. If taken together with

'mauby' which is a tropical drink from buck thorn tree bark.

14. *Raw cacao* is rich in flavonoids and many other anti-inflammatory nutrients found to be useful in lowering the blood pressure. It helps in dealing best with stress. The presence of flavonoids in cacao has been found to provide protection against heart disease and stroke.

15. *Turmeric* which is also known as curcumin has been found to be beneficial in maintaining healthy blood flow, reducing high blood pressure and provides protection from hypercholesterolemia. It is also a natural blood thinner and if taken with black pepper it can work wonders for the health of the heart.

16. *Agathosma betulina* belongs to the family of rutaceae and its common name is buchu is a medicinal plant from South Africa and has been used for centuries by indigenous people to treat many diseases. This herb has been found to be beneficial in reducing high blood pressure naturally.

17. The leaf extract of the plant of *prickly custard apple* has been reported to be beneficial in lowering an elevated blood pressure.

18. *Guan Mu Tong* is a Chinese plant whose extract has been known to possess properties to reduce hypertension.

19. *Breadfruit* plant's leaf extract has been found to lower high blood pressure.

20. *Whole oats* help in reducing hypertension. Eating of whole oats regularly brings significant decrease in blood pressure naturally.

21. *Plantago* supplements can also modestly lower the blood pressure.

22. Regular consumption of *green tea* lowers the blood pressure naturally.

23. A shrub named *'Lasaf'* found in rocky areas at times hanging from the cliffs has been used to produce crude extract that helps in lowering the blood pressure naturally.

24. *Chaksu plant* is usually found in the tropics and has been linked to lower the blood pressure naturally through intravenous use but still we need to know how it works through oral intake.

25. *Coffee weed* is a tree whose leaves are being used for medicinal purpose to lower the blood pressure naturally.

26.   *Black beans* are also known to lower hypertension naturally.

27.   *Karpurvali* also possesses pharmacological properties to lower the blood pressure naturally.

28.   *Virginia dayflower,* a plant native to Southeastern United States has been used in the whole form to get extraction which is reported to decrease high blood pressure.

29.   *River Lily or Swamp lily* has traditionally been used in Western Nigeria to extract its beneficial properties that are being used to lower blood pressure naturally.

30.   *Giant dodder's* crude extract has been reported to bring reduction in blood pressure.

31.   *Carrots* are also known to reduce hypertension naturally.

32.   *Osbeck* – a preparation from dry leaves and stem may also be used to bring reduction in blood pressure.

33.   Eating *oranges* may be beneficial.

34.   *Soybean* has been effective as a hypotensive agent and helps in lowering the blood pressure naturally.

35.   *Pima cotton* is a perennial plant that is native to tropical region which produces black seeds and yellow

flowers. The leaf extract from the plant has been found to be beneficial in reducing the blood pressure.

36.   *Roselle* has been extensively researched for its anti-hypertensive properties. The corolla, calyx and leaves of the plant have been used for medicinal purposes traditionally in many West African countries. It also has been found to lower blood pressure naturally.

37.   Crude extract of *French Lavender* has also been reported to lower hypertension.

38.   *Rompepiedra* also called Stone breaker has been a folk medicine of the Canary Islands and found to possess anti-hypertensive properties.

39.   *Flax seeds* also known as linseed is native to Egypt which is an annual herb and is known to lower blood pressure naturally.

40.   *Black mangrove* is a small tree native to India. The plant's aqueous acetone extract of the plant has been reported to possess antihypertensive properties.

41.   Extract of *tomatoes* contain carotenoids such as vitamin E, beta carotene, and possess antioxidant properties. It also has been found to be beneficial in lowering the blood pressure naturally.

42.   *Murungai's* crude extract has been found to lower blood pressure.

43.   *Umbrella tree* also known as Cork Wood is a plant that grows rapidly and is native to the tropical rainforest area of West Africa. The leaf extract of the plant has been found to lower blood pressure naturally.

44.   Eating *basil* can also lower your blood pressure naturally.

45.   *Harmal* and its crude extract also possess antihypertensive properties.

46.   *Nela nelli plant* has been used traditionally in medicinal practice to lower blood pressure naturally.

47.   *Maritime Pine bark* to extract pycnogenol has been known to modestly reduce hypertension.

48.   *Kudzu plants dry roots* are being used to treat high blood pressure in China.

49.   *Pomegranate* is also known to lower blood pressure naturally.

50.   *Sesame seeds* also help in lowering blood pressure naturally.

Many other natural remedies for the treatment of hypertension may include wheat bran, black plum, ginger, cinnamon, rosemary, stinging nettle, onion, olives, oregano, cardamom, angelica root, ashwagandha root, barley grass, bilberry, black seed oil, cleavers, codonopsis, coleus, forskohlii, corydalis, dandelion roots, hibiscus, hyssop, jiaogulan, lemon, maitake mushroom, mistletoe, motjerwort, passion flower, periwinkle, reishi mushroom, yarrow, ylang-ylang, aloe vera, red clover, saffron, asparagus, lime blossom, olive leave extract, goldenrod, coleus, black cohosh, celery seeds, dashen, cats claw, triphala, jatamansi, arjuna, salmon, dark chocolate, low fat milk, bananas, sweet potatoes, etc.

6. CHAPTER VI. RISK FACTORS ASSOCIATED WITH HIGH BLOOD PRESSURE.

Uncontrolled high blood pressure can lead to many chronic diseases which may include heart failure, stroke, heart attack, dementia, kidney diseases, eye problems, etc. Controlling of high blood pressure is needed to staying healthy and lessening your chances of developing many serious health problems.

Most common risk factor associated with stroke is constant high blood pressure which can cause a break in the weakened blood vessels leading to bleeding in the brain. Blood clot blocking the arteries which are narrow may cause stroke.

High blood pressure can cause bursting or bleeding of the blood vessels of the eyes with the result the vision may be impaired or blurred which could eventually lead to blindness.

With the process of aging and high blood pressure, the arteries usually get hardened throughout the body especially the ones in the brain, heart and kidneys which makes the heart and kidneys to work harder due to the stiffness of arteries.

Our kidneys work as filters to relieve the body of the body waste and toxins. Due to the thickened blood vessels owing to the aging process may leads to high blood pressure and kidneys reduced ability to filter more fluids, consequently the waste starts to accumulate in the body which may lead to the build-up of toxic waste inside the body and may progress to kidney failure. At this point the dialysis or kidney transplant may be needed.

High blood pressure may lead to heart attack and to congestive heart failure if necessary precautionary measure and most needed treatments are being ignored. Arteries are supposed to bring oxygen rich blood to the heart so that the heart gets enough oxygen. If the heart is unable to get enough oxygen you may start feeling chest pain which is commonly referred to as 'angina' and if the flow is totally blocked then a heart attack may result.

Congestive heart failure may be the result of high blood pressure and the heart becomes unable to supply the body of its most needed quantity of oxygen as it is unable to pump out enough blood to carry its function normally.

High blood pressure has the capacity to quietly keep on damaging your body with time without any known symptoms for a long time. If left untreated and uncontrolled may become life threatening and may lead to poor quality of life, disability and heart attack which could prove to be fatal. There can be many complications and one may lead to the next problem therefore timely precautionary measures needed to be taken and if diagnosed with hypertension then it becomes very important to keep it controlled at all times and in all conditions.

7. CHAPTER VII. PREVENTION OF HYPERTENSION

Lifestyle changes may be recommended to lay foundations for preventive measures and lower the chances of its occurrence. Following are few of the points that needed consideration.

• Reduce the dietary food sources of salt.

• Maintain your ideal body weight according to your height.

• Increase your physical activity.

• Limit your alcohol consumption.

• Consume a diet rich in fresh fruits, whole grain cereals, nuts, seeds, legumes, beans, pulses and vegetables.

• Make use of fresh or powdered garlic.

• Eat fish at least twice a week.

• Consume milk and milk products regularly.

• Learn the techniques of managing your stress and anxiety level.

• Avoid smoking.

• Limit your intake of caffeine containing beverages.

8. CHAPTER VIII. DASH DIET FOR HYPERTENSION

Dash has been known to be helpful in reducing high blood pressure in just 14 days. You do not even have to lower your salt intake in this and it is easy to follow. This kind of diet is being recommended to newly diagnosed cases of hypertension.

This diet can help in reducing medication and in pre-hypertensive and moderately high blood pressure cases it can even help in eliminating the medications. This diet is rich in minerals such as calcium, potassium and magnesium and is beneficial in lowering the blood pressure. It has been noted that the supplements of the same mineral do not have the same effect as the diet, there is something in the diet in addition to these minerals that aids in bringing the blood pressure to the normal range.

Dash diet is based on nuts, fruits, vegetables, seeds, legumes, lean meat, low fat dairy, fish, poultry, and whole grain cereals. This diet has been found to be beneficial in lowering serum cholesterol, reducing insulin resistance and increasing weight loss. In addition to dash diet you must try to restrict your salt intake and wherever possible omit its use.

9. CHAPTER IX.
ALTERNATIVE TREATMENTS

In addition to medication, adhere to the dash diet which will help in keeping your blood pressure in check. You can also avail the option of many available alternative therapies such as stress reduction through breathing techniques, herbal treatment, natural therapy, use of supplementation, acupuncture, etc. Through research studies we have come to know that many of these alternative therapies can work well, sometimes in isolation and other times in addition to the conventional method of treatment. Most of these alternative therapies are quite safe to use and possess a capacity to work wonders.

Breathing Technique – Emotional stress can lead to high blood pressure and managing the stress level properly aids in reducing the blood pressure. Some of the alternative therapies that could be used effectively to lower the blood pressure may include oigong, tai chi, yoga, slow breathing, etc.

*Oigong*_promotes relaxation through a combination of movement and deep breathing techniques.

Tai chi is a popular alternative treatment method used for relaxation and fitness purposes. It is gentle with stretching movements and flowing exercises.

Yoga is being used to improve and enhance body circulation and flexibility which results in overall sense of wellbeing. Great cardiovascular beneficial aspects are attached with yoga through the means of stretching exercises and breathing techniques. It helps in increasing flexibility, fitness and strength and provides a technique for relaxation.

Slow breathing for at least 15 minutes on a daily basis can help in lowering blood pressure within three months' time.

Herbal therapy could be used to natural lower the blood pressure. Many herbs are known for their blood pressure lowering action through studies as well as trial and error basis. Besides blood pressure lowering action, many also contribute towards better and improved overall circulation system such as garlic, hibiscus and hawthorn.

Many known *supplements* also provide an option of alternative therapy and play a part in lowering the blood pressure such as co enzyme Q10, Omega-3 fatty acids, etc.

Acupuncture is more alternative therapy to lower blood pressure naturally and you need to discuss with your doctor before you take any decision regarding an alternative therapy.

Use of *aromatherapy* using several *essential oils* has also proved to be beneficial in reducing the stress level.

10. CHAPTER X. CONCLUSION

So now we can conclusively say that many unnecessary deaths occurring worldwide due to hypertension, and many diseases which are the result of this problematic health condition, we need to take preventive measures not only on an individual level but also on a community as well as on the national level to overcome it in a global form.

Prevention has always proved to be highly beneficial in comparison to cure not only just for an individual but for bringing worldwide betterment in improvement in overall health and wellbeing.

With the onset of hypertension, both preventive measures as well as treatment methods may be needed. Consult your physician for the best medication or combination of medication that may suit you best and opt for a dash diet which will help in keeping it under control.

Your doctor may be the best available guide for you who may support or reject any idea of alternative treatment in addition to a medical treatment in the light of all the available medical reports and your overall health condition.

You must in all circumstances take good care of yourself, eat right kind of diet, follow right type of sleeping pattern, disconnect with all wrong health deteriorating habits and learn to relax and give rest to your mind as the whole body system is connected with the brain system. Any irregularity or irresponsibility towards our brain may start to show sign and symptoms of body malfunction.

Learn to adapt and simplify things for yourself in order to have peace of mind. Wisdom to de clutter and living a more natural life show a path of relaxation, happiness and peace. Believe in the basics of life because you are the most important entity for yourself.

Know your limits in regards to achievements as we all crave to keep achieving but we have to be more realistic towards our approach to what is accessible with ease and what is accessible with disease.

Have faith in yourself than faith in the material world. We all have seen that running after the material goods, all around the world has only been able to give us the stress, anxiety, depression and unhappiness. There are innumerable benefits attached with many material goods, only if these could be achieved with health giving factors and not vice versa.

Try to avoid salt in the diet and whenever possible try to replace these with the aromas of natural food ingredients, spices and herbs. A little sprinkle of many irresistible herbs and healthy spices may give better taste, flavor and aroma than with added salt. Look for the options and be more creative in your recipe adaptations. Develop new recipes to suit your health requirements and follow a dash diet.

Get at least 6 to 8 hours undisturbed sleep. For good sleep you may make use of hair massage oil with a suitable essential oil and massage this oil on your head before sleeping. Next morning when you will wake up you may feel relaxed and with renewed energy.

Your brain is a concentrated form of fat. It is mainly composed of fats and it loves the energy of fats through massage. Give the energy that your mind needs and you will find that you are better able to fight with stress and stress giving factors.

Learn the techniques of deep breathing and breathe deeply for at least 15 minutes daily. You may be able to reduce your blood pressure without any medications. Look for the causes and try to eliminate these through better alternatives. Instead of smoking try aromatherapy that may help you in quitting this health destructing factor and habit.

Have faith in your will power and deal with all the causes one by one so that you do not start feeling deprived of the many good things that you have to give away. A dash diet is not a very strict type of diet and you are able to enjoy many food items. Try to consume more plant based foods and increase your physical activity. If you feel you are unable to take out time for gym you may always try to increase your activity through other means. Be more active means be less lazy. Have more outdoor activities as gardening, walking, etc.

Spend less time in front of T.V and computer and more with humans so that you get the essence of life and find natural means of relaxation. Be more creative and productive so that you may find peace of mind in just simple things.

You do not have to reach the top of Mount Everest to find peace, relaxation and stress free life. It may be lying just next to you and you only need to be aware of what good help you what bad punish you.

Quit smoking, limit your alcohol consumption and lead a more beneficial, successful and happy life through means of nature and natural therapies. Do not work so hard and so much that you forget yourself and your existence. Give more time to yourself and your personal needs so that the doors of stress never find you. Happiness comes from within and happiness is the foundation of good health.

Be happy and contented with yourself and your life in general. There is no perfect world and you will never be able to find one. Change what you easily can and try to communicate the idea of what you cannot but do believe in. Understand yourself better and know your needs. Fulfill all your basic needs in the right and healthy manner to achieve long lasting health, happiness and success. Do great things and live a great life, but only in simple manner.